Rhabdomyolysis

The Ultimate Guide to clinical manifestations and complications

Dr. Robert Neil

Table of Content

Introduction

The disease known as rhabdomyolysis is characterized by the disintegration of muscle fibers and the subsequent discharge of their contents into the circulation. Serious side effects such as electrolyte imbalances and renal failure may result from this. Among the clinical signs of rhabdomyolysis are:

- tenderness, edema, and soreness in the muscles.
- Urine that is brown or dark red.
- experiencing weakness or exhaustion, making it difficult to finish workouts or job duties.
- Unexpectedly acute aches, pains, or cramps in the muscles.
- Disorientation, dehydration, fever, vomiting, nausea, vomiting, and lack of consciousness.

The following are the primary rhabdomyolysis complications:

1. Acute renal failure: The distal convoluted tubules can produce a myoglobin cast, renal

vasoconstriction, and ischemia can all cause this.

2. Electrolyte disorders: Common conditions include early hypocalcemia, late hypercalcemia, hyperphosphatemia, and hyperkalemia.

3. Metabolic acidosis: This condition may be brought on by the poisonous compounds that injured muscles release.

4. Compartmental syndrome: This condition can develop when fluid builds up in a closed bodily compartment, which can cause pain and increased pressure.
5. Disseminated intravascular coagulopathy: a potentially fatal consequence that can result in aberrant blood clot development all over the body.

Early intervention is necessary for rhabdomyolysis recovery. Drink plenty of water, get plenty of rest, and stay out of the heat if the condition is mild. Intravenous (IV) fluids, hospitalization, and close observation for irregular cardiac rhythms, impaired kidney function, convulsions, raised compartment pressures, and elevated potassium levels may be necessary in moderate to severe cases. A better prognosis and a full recovery without side effects can result from early diagnosis and treatment.

chapter One

Causes of Rhabdomyolysis

Numerous conditions, such as direct muscle injury, overexertion, heat exposure, drug toxicity, metabolic problems, infections, electrolyte imbalances, genetic diseases, and extended bed rest, can result in rhabdomyolysis. Rhabdomyolysis is frequently caused by trauma, including crush injuries, falls, and building collapses. Third-degree burns, lightning strikes, and electrical shock injuries are additional physical causes. Rhabdomyolysis can result from non-physical factors such as alcoholism or drug abuse, such as using heroin, cocaine, or amphetamines. Rhabdomyolysis is also frequently caused by severe muscle tension, viral myositis, connective tissue diseases, and drug overdose. Rhabdomyolysis in the workplace can result from direct injuries, physical activity, and heat exposure. In order to avoid severe consequences such as disseminated intravascular coagulopathy, metabolic acidosis, acute renal failure, electrolyte imbalances, and compartmental syndrome, prompt treatment is crucial.

1.1 Trauma and Injury

Less than 20 percent of cases of rhabdomyolysis are caused by trauma or injury. Rhabdomyolysis can result from traumatic traumas such as falls, crush injuries, and building collapses. Rhabdomyolysis can also result after lightning strikes, electrical shock injuries, and third-degree burns. Rhabdomyolysis can also result from physical compression, such as that which occurs after extended immobilization following a fall. Rhabdomyolysis in the workplace can result from direct injuries, physical activity, and heat exposure. The degree of muscle injury and the quantity of myoglobin and other muscle components discharged into the bloodstream determine the severity of rhabdomyolysis. Rhabdomyolysis can cause muscle soreness, dark urine, weakness, and, in more severe cases, consequences such as disseminated intravascular coagulopathy, acute renal failure, metabolic acidosis, electrolyte abnormalities, and compartmental syndrome. Early intervention is necessary to avoid major health issues and improve the likelihood of a speedy recovery.

1.2 Medications and Toxins

The disease known as rhabdomyolysis is characterized by the disintegration of skeletal muscle tissue, which allows myoglobin to be released into the circulation. Both drugs and poisons have the potential to aggravate rhabdomyolysis's clinical symptoms and raise the possibility of consequences.

1. Drugs Linked to Rhabdomyolysis: *Statins*: Medicines that decrease cholesterol, such as statins, can occasionally damage muscles, particularly when taken in larger dosages.

*Fibrates:*Fibrates are a different class of lipid-lowering drugs that have been associated with rhabdomyolysis, especially when taken in conjunction with statins.

Antipsychotics: Antipsychotic drugs, including olanzapine and clozapine, have the potential to exacerbate muscle injury.

Antibiotics:A number of medications, such as macrolides and fluoroquinolones, have been linked to cases of rhabdomyolysis.

2. Toxins and Rhabdomyolysis:
Alcohol: Drinking too much alcohol can cause rhabdomyolysis and the disintegration of muscles.

Illicit Drugs: Drugs like amphetamines and cocaine can cause rhabdomyolysis, frequently as a result of decreased blood supply and increased muscle activity.

Venoms: Toxins introduced by snake and insect bites might cause rhabdomyolysis.

3. Clinical Manifestations:
Muscle Weakness and Pain: Severe muscle pain and weakness are frequently seen in the early stages of the illness.

Dark Urine: Patients may have dark, reddish-brown urine due to the presence of myoglobin. Fatigue and malaise: Patients may feel generally tired and lethargic.

4. Rhabdomyolysis Complications:
Acute Kidney Injury (AKI): Myoglobin produced from injured muscles can harm the kidneys, which can result in AKI.

Electrolyte Imbalances: Intracellular substances can leak out, upsetting the electrolyte balance and perhaps leading to fatal consequences.

Compartment Syndrome: Severe cases may result in compartment syndrome, a condition in which increased pressure from swollen muscles affects blood flow.

5. Management and Treatment:
Fluid Resuscitation: By flushing away myoglobin and preserving proper hydration, intravenous fluids are essential to preventing kidney injury.

Monitoring Electrolytes: To effectively manage problems, electrolyte levels must be regularly monitored.

Identifying and Withdrawing Causative Agents: A crucial component of treatment is stopping prescription drugs or taking care of toxin exposure.
Healthcare practitioners must comprehend the connection between drugs, toxins, and rhabdomyolysis in order to quickly diagnose and treat this potentially dangerous disorder. Early intervention can lower the risk of complications and have a major impact on patient outcomes.

1.3 Metabolic Disorders

The disease known as rhabdomyolysis is defined by the disintegration of skeletal muscle tissue and the subsequent leakage of muscle cell contents into the circulation. Rhabdomyolysis can arise as a result of metabolic diseases, which can further exacerbate its consequences and clinical signs.

1. Triggers for Metabolism:
Rhabdomyolysis can be triggered by metabolic abnormalities such as metabolic myopathies or disruptions in the metabolism of fats and carbohydrates. Deviations from these metabolic pathways weaken the integrity of muscle cells and make them more vulnerable to injury.

2. Clinical Manifestations: *Weakness and Pain in the Muscles:* Because rhabdomyolysis causes muscle cell breakdown, significant muscle discomfort and weakening are common presentations.

Dull Pee: Urine that is dark and tea-colored, indicative of myoglobinuria, can be produced when injured muscles release myoglobin.

3. Difficulties: *Injury to the kidneys (AKI)*: Renal tubular blockage brought on by myoglobin produced during rhabdomyolysis may result in AKI. It is essential to act quickly to stop kidney damage.
Imbalances in Electrolytes: Electrolyte imbalances caused by the release of intracellular materials, such as potassium, can

result in cardiac arrhythmias and other problems.

4. Diagnostic Challenges - Laboratory Investigations: Rhabdomyolysis raises the level of creatine kinase (CK); however, further testing, such as genetic analysis or a metabolic profile, may be necessary to uncover underlying metabolic problems.

Clinical History: Correct diagnosis and efficient treatment depend on an understanding of a patient's metabolic history.

5. Fluid Resuscitation: *Treatment Strategies*: Staying well hydrated is crucial for preventing renal problems since it facilitates the removal of myoglobin from the kidneys.

Taking Care of Underlying Disorders: Treatment options for metabolic diseases that cause rhabdomyolysis include food changes, medication, and other focused interventions.

6. Long-Term Considerations: *Preventive Measures*: Individuals with metabolic diseases

that are known to put them at risk for rhabdomyolysis should take preventive steps, such as taking the right medication and changing their lifestyle.

Watching: To identify and treat repeated episodes and reduce the risk of consequences, long-term monitoring is essential.

In conclusion, the interaction between rhabdomyolysis and metabolic problems highlights the significance of a thorough approach to diagnosis, treatment, and prevention that addresses underlying metabolic abnormalities in addition to acute symptoms.

Chapter Two

Pathophysiology of Muscle Breakdown

A complicated medical disorder known as rhabdomyolysis causes skeletal muscle that has been wounded or damaged to dissolve quickly, releasing intracellular components of the muscle into the bloodstream and extracellular space. These components include myoglobin, creatine kinase, aldolase, and electrolytes. Rhabdomyolysis can be brought on by any type of direct or indirect muscular injury. Trauma is frequently caused by falls, crush injuries, electrical shock injuries, building collapses, and third-degree burns, among other key contributing factors. Furthermore, severe muscle strain, medication toxicity, infections, and metabolic abnormalities are examples of nontraumatic causes. Rhabdomyolysis's systemic effects can result in consequences such as disseminated intravascular coagulopathy, acute renal failure, metabolic acidosis, electrolyte abnormalities, and compartmental syndrome. In order to avoid significant medical issues and improve the likelihood of a speedy recovery, prompt treatment is necessary.

2.1 Muscle Fiber Damage

Rhabdomyolysis-Related Muscle Fiber Damage: Clinical Signs and Outcomes.

A complicated medical disorder known as rhabdomyolysis causes damaged or injured muscle fibers to dissolve quickly and leak their contents into the bloodstream. Numerous problems, some potentially fatal, may result from this condition

- Risk factors and causes

Numerous factors can lead to rhabdomyolysis, such as:

i. Crush or trauma wounds
ii. Addiction to substances like PCP, heroin, amphetamines, cocaine, or statins
iii. Genetic disorders of the muscles
iv. Abrupt changes in body temperature
v. Low phosphate levels Muscle tissue

vi. Prolonged surgical operations; seizures or tremors in the muscles; severe exertion, including marathon running or calisthenics; severe dehydration.

- Clinical Indications

Rhabdomyolysis can present with a variety of clinical signs; however, some typical ones are as follows:

Weakness, stiffness, and discomfort in the muscles.

deep, scarlet, or coke-purple color;

weakness and aches in the muscles

Stooling and queasiness

High fever and tachycardia

Bewilderment, thirst, and unconsciousness.

- Difficulties

Rhabdomyolysis can cause serious complications, which can include:

1. Acute tubular necrosis: Toxic chemicals released from muscle fibers cause damage to the kidney tubules.

2. Acute renal failure: kidney failure brought on by ischemia, myoglobin cast formation in the distal convoluted tubules, and renal vasoconstriction.

3. Dangerous chemical imbalances in the blood: Hyperphosphatemia, early hypocalcemia, late hypercalcemia, and hyperkalemia are examples of electrolyte disorders that can cause major issues with the heart and other organs.

4. Shock (low blood pressure): Muscle fibers can release toxins that can result in hypotension, which can then cause shock.

5. Compartmental syndrome: Pain, edema, and impaired blood flow may result from increased pressure inside a closed fascial compartment.

6. Disseminated intravascular coagulopathy: abnormal blood clotting may result from myoglobin released into the bloodstream.

- Preventive and Therapeutic Measures

Staying hydrated, avoiding overexertion, and avoiding potential causes are the three main ways to prevent rhabdomyolysis. It is imperative that you get medical help as soon as you suspect rhabdomyolysis because prompt diagnosis and treatment can greatly enhance the prognosis and lower the risk of complications. Dialysis, medicine, intravenous fluids, and surgery are possible treatment options.

2.2 Release of Myoglobin into the Bloodstream

A dangerous medical disorder known as rhabdomyolysis is defined by the disintegration of muscle tissue and the subsequent release of the contents of the muscle fiber, including the protein myoglobin, into the bloodstream. Serious side effects from this illness include kidney failure, abnormal heartbeats, and even death. When muscle tissue is harmed, myoglobin is released into the bloodstream, which can be harmful to the kidneys and other organs.

The following clinical symptoms and consequences may arise from myoglobin leakage into the bloodstream:

1. Myalgias: Rhabdomyolysis frequently manifests as stiffness and soreness in the muscles.

2. Muscle weakness: myoglobin leakage into the bloodstream and possible muscle injury may be indicated by this.

3. Red to brown urine: Because myoglobin is present in the urine, myoglobinuria might result in red to brown urine.

4. Electrolyte imbalances: High blood levels of potassium, sodium, and other electrolytes as a result of rhabdomyolysis might result in irregular heartbeats and other problems.

5. Kidney failure: Kidney failure can result from damage to the kidneys caused by the leakage of myoglobin and other muscle contents into the bloodstream.

6. Problems with bleeding and clotting: Rhabdomyolysis may result in problems with bleeding and clotting, which raises the possibility of complications.

7. Compartment syndrome: This excruciating ailment arises from an increase in pressure within a muscle group and can exacerbate pre-existing muscle damage.

To avoid potentially fatal consequences and improve the prognosis for a full recovery, it is imperative to identify and treat rhabdomyolysis as soon as possible. Depending on the patient's underlying medical issues and the severity of the illness, treatment options may include dialysis, medication, intravenous fluids, or surgery. It's critical to get medical aid as soon as you suspect rhabdomyolysis because prompt care can help avoid serious consequences and improve the prognosis.

<h1 style="text-align:center">Chapter Three</h1>

Clinical Manifestations

Myalgia, weakness, and myoglobinuria are the three symptoms that define rhabdomyolysis; the most sensitive test for this condition is an increase in creatine kinase (CK) levels. Less than 10% of patients exhibit the traditional trio; hence, those with established risk factors—such as trauma, infection, muscle illness, and immobilization—should be suspected of having rhabdomyolysis. Additional typical indications and manifestations of rhabdomyolysis encompass reddish-brown urine, weakened muscles, pain in the shoulders, thighs, or lower back, stomach discomfort, emesis, fever, a fast heartbeat, and disorientation. Acute renal failure, electrolyte imbalances, compartment syndrome, and disseminated intravascular coagulopathy are other consequences associated with rhabdomyolysis.

Early diagnosis and treatment are essential to avoid serious complications like kidney failure, an irregular heartbeat, and even death; thus, it's critical to detect the symptoms and signs of rhabdomyolysis as soon as possible. Seeking medical assistance right away is recommended if rhabdomyolysis is suspected in order to start appropriate management and avoid potentially fatal consequences.

3.1 Signs and Symptoms

A medical disorder called rhabdomyolysis can present with a variety of symptoms. Myalgia, weakness, and myoglobinuria make up the traditional triad of symptoms; the most sensitive test is an increase in creatine kinase (CK) levels. Less than 10% of patients exhibit the traditional trio; hence, those with established risk factors—such as trauma, infection, muscle illness, and immobilization—should be suspected of having rhabdomyolysis. Additional typical indications and manifestations of rhabdomyolysis encompass reddish-brown urine, weakened muscles, pain in the shoulders, thighs, or lower back, stomach discomfort, emesis, fever, a fast heartbeat, and disorientation. Acute renal failure, electrolyte imbalances, compartment syndrome, and disseminated intravascular coagulopathy are other consequences associated with rhabdomyolysis.

It's critical to identify rhabdomyolysis symptoms and signs as soon as possible since severe problems, including kidney failure, abnormal heartbeats, and even death, can be avoided with early diagnosis and treatment. Seeking medical assistance right away is recommended if rhabdomyolysis is suspected in order to start appropriate management and avoid potentially fatal consequences.

Depending on the severity of the ailment and the underlying cause, rhabdomyolysis can induce a variety of other signs and symptoms in addition to the typical triad. For instance, the patient may have fever, itching, and a skin rash if the illness is the result of a medication reaction. The patient may have flu-like symptoms, such as fever, headache, and muscular aches, if the illness is brought on by a viral infection. Rhabdomyolysis can result in a coma, seizures, and even death in extreme situations.

It's crucial to remember that some rhabdomyolysis individuals may not exhibit any symptoms at all, particularly if the underlying cause is not severe or the illness is mild. Consequently, even in the absence of symptoms, it is crucial to seek medical assistance if any of the risk factors for rhabdomyolysis—such as trauma, infection, muscle illness, and immobilization—are present.

In conclusion, rhabdomyolysis can result in a variety of symptoms, such as red to dark urine, muscle soreness, abdominal discomfort, nausea, vomiting, fever, a fast heartbeat, disorientation, and more. The traditional triad of myalgia, weakness, and myoglobinuria can also be caused by this condition. To avoid serious consequences and enhance the prognosis, it is imperative to identify and treat rhabdomyolysis as soon as possible.

3.2 Diagnostic Criteria

A combination of imaging scans, laboratory testing, and clinical signs and symptoms are used to diagnose rhabdomyolysis. Less than 10% of patients exhibit the traditional triad of rhabdomyolysis symptoms, which include myalgia, weakness, and tea-colored urine. Consequently, rhabdomyolysis should be suspected in any patient who has a known risk factor, such as trauma, infection, muscle illness, or immobilization. The most sensitive test for rhabdomyolysis, serum creatine kinase (CK) levels, may indicate the presence of an indirect clue, such as muscle injury accompanied by an unexpected increase in CK levels.

Serum CK levels, which are typically raised, and urine testing for myoglobin, a byproduct of muscle breakdown that can harm the kidneys, are two laboratory tests for rhabdomyolysis. Imaging tests, such as computed tomography (CT) and magnetic resonance imaging (MRI), can also be performed to determine the extent of muscle damage and rule out other medical disorders that might be causing the same symptoms.

Because severe disease can result in an accumulation of nitrogenous products in the blood (azotemia), with or without a loss in renal function and electrolyte abnormalities, prompt detection and treatment of rhabdomyolysis are essential. Thus, it is imperative to seek medical assistance as soon as rhabdomyolysis is detected in order to commence effective management and avoid potentially fatal consequences.

Chapter Four

Diagnosis and Evaluation

A thorough method is used in the diagnosis and assessment of rhabdomyolysis in order to determine the underlying cause, gauge the extent of muscle damage, and find any possible consequences. A comprehensive patient history that includes recent trauma, exertion, drug use, and medical disorders, in addition to clinical signs including muscle soreness, weakness, and black urine, might offer crucial diagnostic hints. In order to diagnose and assess issues related to rhabdomyolysis, laboratory testing is essential. Serum creatine kinase (CK), myoglobin, electrolytes, and renal function can all be measured. Compartment syndrome and myoglobinuria can be assessed by imaging techniques such as urinalysis and compartment pressure measurements. Furthermore, the proper management and treatment of problems such as disseminated intravascular coagulopathy, acute renal failure, metabolic acidosis, and electrolyte imbalances depend on their identification. Initiating appropriate therapies and preventing potential bad outcomes associated with rhabdomyolysis require a precise and quick diagnosis.

4.1 Laboratory Tests (Creatine Kinase, Myoglobin)

A thorough method is used in the diagnosis and assessment of rhabdomyolysis in order to determine the underlying cause, gauge the extent of muscle damage, and find any possible consequences. A comprehensive patient history that includes recent trauma, exertion, drug use, and medical disorders, in addition to clinical signs including muscle soreness, weakness, and black urine, might offer crucial diagnostic hints. In order to diagnose and assess issues related to rhabdomyolysis, laboratory testing is essential. Serum creatine kinase (CK), myoglobin, electrolytes, and renal function can all be measured.

Serum creatine kinase (CK) levels: CK is a crucial indicator of muscle injury and is usually markedly increased in cases of rhabdomyolysis. Although the absolute number does not always indicate the severity of the problem, there may be a correlation between the degree of CK increase and the severity of muscle injury.

Myoglobin: Found in both blood and urine, myoglobin is a protein that is liberated from injured muscle cells. Myoglobinemia, or high blood levels of the protein, and myoglobinuria, or the presence of myoglobin in the urine, are signs of muscle injury and can lead to the development of problems such as acute renal failure.

Tests for electrolytes, specifically potassium, phosphorus, and calcium, as well as tests for renal function, including blood urea nitrogen (BUN) and serum creatinine, are crucial for assessing and keeping an eye out for complications like acute renal failure and electrolyte imbalances.

Compartment syndrome and myoglobinuria can be assessed by imaging techniques such as urinalysis and compartment pressure measurements. Furthermore, the proper management and treatment of problems such as disseminated intravascular coagulopathy, acute renal failure, metabolic acidosis, and electrolyte imbalances depend on their identification. Initiating appropriate therapies and preventing potential bad outcomes associated with rhabdomyolysis require a precise and quick diagnosis.

4.2 Imaging Studies

In cases of rhabdomyolysis, imaging tests typically have limited diagnostic use. However, radiography might be taken into consideration in particular situations, such as suspected fractures. The history, physical examination, and laboratory tests—such as myoglobin measures and serum creatine kinase (CK) levels—are the main components of the clinical diagnosis of rhabdomyolysis. Depending on the underlying etiology, imaging results for rhabdomyolysis can show evidence of bleeding or edema in the muscles. Imaging tests are useful in determining the extent of muscle injury and in evaluating concomitant disorders such as compartment syndrome, even though they may not be routinely used to diagnose rhabdomyolysis. In order to determine the most effective management and treatment plans, the major diagnostic strategy for rhabdomyolysis continues to be centered on clinical and laboratory evaluation.

4.3 Differential Diagnosis

A high index of suspicion and a thorough approach are necessary for the diagnosis of rhabdomyolysis in order to determine the underlying etiology, evaluate the extent of muscle damage, and identify any potential consequences. Differential diagnosis is crucial since the clinical signs of rhabdomyolysis are nonspecific and can resemble those of other illnesses. In addition to polymyositis, dermatomyositis, viral myositis, and metabolic myopathies, other disorders that might cause muscle discomfort, weakness, and dark urine are listed. Myoglobin measures and serum creatine kinase (CK) levels are two crucial laboratory tests for diagnosing and evaluating rhabdomyolysis. Compartment syndrome and myoglobinuria can be assessed by imaging techniques such as urinalysis and compartment pressure measurements. Furthermore, the proper management and treatment of problems such as disseminated intravascular coagulopathy, acute renal failure, metabolic acidosis, and electrolyte imbalances depend on their identification. Important diagnostic hints can be obtained from a thorough patient history that includes recent trauma, physical activity, drug use, and medical disorders. Initiating appropriate therapies and preventing potential unfavorable consequences associated with rhabdomyolysis require a precise and quick diagnosis.

Chapter Five

Complications Associated with Rhabdomyolysis

Acute renal failure, metabolic acidosis, disseminated intravascular coagulopathy, compartmental syndrome, and electrolyte imbalances are just a few of the problems that can arise from the complicated medical illness known as rhabdomyolysis.

One of the most frequent and dangerous side effects of rhabdomyolysis is acute renal failure, which is brought on by myoglobin buildup in the renal tubules and causes myoglobin cast formation, ischemia, and renal vasoconstriction.

Rhabdomyolysis can also result in electrolyte imbalances, which can cause cardiac arrhythmias, seizures, and neuromuscular dysfunction. These imbalances can include hyperkalemia, hyperphosphatemia, early hypocalcemia, and late hypercalcemia. When poisonous compounds are released from injured muscles, it can cause metabolic acidosis, which lowers bicarbonate and pH levels.

Increased pressure and pain can result from fluid buildup in a closed bodily compartment, which can cause compartmental syndrome. A potentially fatal consequence of disseminated intravascular coagulopathy is the production of aberrant blood clots all over the body. Initiating appropriate therapies and preventing potential unfavorable consequences associated with rhabdomyolysis require a precise and quick diagnosis.

5.1 Acute Kidney Injury

Rhabdomyolysis can cause acute kidney damage (AKI), a dangerous side effect that affects 33% to 50% of patients.

Numerous variables, such as hypovolemia, medications, dehydration, hypoperfusion, and pigment-induced distal tube injury, are linked to the development of AKI in rhabdomyolysis. Patients with creatine kinase (CK) levels above 40,000 IU/L are at an increased risk of developing AKI.

Rhabdomyolysis-related AKI clinical symptoms include.

Hypertension, Pulmonary Edema, Fluid Overload, Oliguria or Anuria, and Congestive Heart Failure

Preventing or treating the condition's principal consequence is the main goal of managing acute kidney injury in rhabdomyolysis. Important facets of management consist of:

1. Fluid management: To reduce the risk of AKI, rhabdomyolysis must be identified and treated as soon as possible. The goal of fluid management is to avoid fluid buildup in muscle compartments, which can exacerbate renal hypoperfusion, and to maintain appropriate hydration.

2. Monitoring and dialysis: The management of AKI in rhabdomyolysis depends on careful observation of renal function and the use of dialysis when required.

3. Identifying and managing underlying causes: In order to lower the risk of AKI, it is critical to recognize and treat the underlying causes of rhabdomyolysis, which include trauma, drug toxicity, infections, and metabolic abnormalities.

Early detection and effective treatment of rhabdomyolysis might help avoid complications such as acute kidney injury (AKI), which can have a major negative effect on patient outcomes.

5.2 Electrolyte Imbalances

Because they can result in a variety of clinical symptoms and consequences, electrolyte imbalances are a serious side effect of rhabdomyolysis.

The following electrolyte imbalances are most frequently linked to rhabdomyolysis:

1. Hyperkalemia: Elevated serum potassium levels can result from rhabdomyolysis, which releases significant amounts of potassium into

the bloodstream from injured muscle cells. Heart arrhythmias, neuromuscular malfunctions, and other potentially fatal consequences can result from hyperkalemia.

2. Hypophosphatemia: Elevations in serum phosphate levels can result from the release of myoglobin and other products of protein breakdown during rhabdomyolysis. Other electrolyte abnormalities, like hypocalcemia and hyperkalemia, can arise as a result of hyperphosphatemia.

3. Hypocalcemia: The release of negatively charged proteins and phospholipids from injured muscle cells during rhabdomyolysis may result in a brief drop in serum calcium levels. Neuromuscular dysfunction, such as paresthesias, seizures, and muscle weakening, can result from hypocalcemia.

4. Metabolic disorders: acidosis, oxidative stress, dehydration, and other metabolic abnormalities can all be brought on by Rhabdomyolysis. Electrolyte imbalances and

other rhabdomyolysis-related problems may arise as a result of these illnesses.

It is imperative to promptly diagnose and treat rhabdomyolysis in order to avoid electrolyte imbalances and other consequences. Treatment approaches that help maintain normal electrolyte levels and enhance patient outcomes include fluid resuscitation, dialysis, and the use of particular electrolyte replenishment products.

5.3. Disseminated Intravascular Coagulation (DIC)

One serious and perhaps fatal side effect of rhabdomyolysis is called disseminated intravascular coagulation (DIC). It is typified by the coagulation system becoming widely activated, which causes blood clots to develop in tiny blood vessels all over the body. The body's platelets and clotting factors may be depleted as a result of this process, which could cause severe bleeding and organ damage.

When rhabdomyolysis occurs, DIC is linked to the bloodstream release of myoglobin and other components of muscle breakdown, which can start the coagulation cascade and cause systemic blood clotting. As a late consequence of rhabdomyolysis, the development of DIC is frequently linked to elevated prothrombin time and activated partial thromboplastin time.

Clinical signs of DIC in rhabdomyolysis can include symptoms including decreased urine output, blood in the stools or urine, bleeding from the nose or gums, and unexplained bruises. Shock and organ failure are possible outcomes of severe cases of DIC.

When DIC is used in conjunction with rhabdomyolysis, the underlying cause must be addressed. This may entail using blood products to support the body's clotting function and vigorous fluid resuscitation to avoid kidney damage. To stop DIC from getting worse and from having related problems, it must be identified and treated as soon as possible.

Chapter Six

Treatment Approaches

The management of rhabdomyolysis's side effects and underlying causes is the main goal of treatment. Preventing acute kidney injury, restoring electrolyte imbalances, and maintaining appropriate fluid resuscitation are the basic objectives of treatment.

- Methods of Treatment:

1. Fluid Resuscitation: Drink enough water to avoid renal injury and to help the bloodstream remove myoglobin and other products of muscle breakdown. Usually, intravenous fluids are given to maintain urine production and shield the kidneys from damage.

2. Determining and Handling Fundamental Reasons: The underlying causes of rhabdomyolysis, such as trauma, drug toxicity, infections, and metabolic abnormalities, must be found and treated. Important components of

treatment include eliminating the causing substances and administering the necessary medical interventions.

3. Monitoring and Correction of Electrolyte Abnormalities: It's important to keep a close eye on the levels of electrolytes, especially calcium, phosphorus, and potassium. To avoid cardiac arrhythmias, muscular weakness, and other issues related to electrolyte imbalances, any abnormalities must be promptly corrected.
4. Preventing Acute Kidney Injury: A vital part of managing rhabdomyolysis is taking steps to prevent acute kidney injury, such as keeping a proper fluid balance and closely monitoring kidney function.

5. Anesthetic concerns: To provide safe perioperative care, special concerns pertaining to the management of rhabdomyolysis and its possible consequences should be taken into account when anesthesia is needed for surgical procedures.

To guarantee thorough therapy and maximize patient outcomes, the treatment of rhabdomyolysis necessitates a multidisciplinary strategy requiring tight collaboration amongst healthcare experts, such as emergency medicine physicians, intensivists, nephrologists, and surgeons.

6.1 Fluid Resuscitation

The mainstay of rhabdomyolysis treatment is fluid resuscitation, which tries to minimize the systemic effects of muscle breakdown and avoid acute renal impairment. Maintaining an appropriate intravascular volume, enhancing renal perfusion, and assisting in the removal of myoglobin and other byproducts of muscle breakdown are the basic objectives of fluid resuscitation.

When performing resuscitation for rhabdomyolysis, fluid selection is crucial. For fluid resuscitation in this situation, both lactated Ringer's solution and regular saline (0.9% or 0.45%) are suitable. Reducing renal vasoconstriction and producing diluted urine is the goal of fluid resuscitation, as this will lessen the amount of myoglobin precipitation.

To sustain a urine output goal of 200 to 300 mL/h, aggressive fluid resuscitation using isotonic fluids, such as normal saline, should be started. This increased flow of urine lowers the risk of kidney damage by preventing the buildup of myoglobin in the renal tubules. Diuretics may be used to increase urine production in situations of severe rhabdomyolysis, but caution should be exercised since they may worsen volume depletion and electrolyte imbalances.

Hemodialysis should be taken into consideration as a therapeutic option when there is metabolic acidosis and life-threatening hyperkalemia. Furthermore, crucial components of treatment for compartmental syndrome include monitoring intra-compartmental pressure and, if necessary, undergoing fasciotomy.

In order to avoid acute kidney damage and other systemic problems linked to rhabdomyolysis, early and vigorous fluid resuscitation using isotonic fluids is a crucial part of the treatment of this illness.

6.2 Electrolyte Management

Since rhabdomyolysis is linked to a number of electrolyte abnormalities, such as hyperkalemia, hypocalcemia, hyperphosphatemia, and hyperuricemia, managing electrolytes is an essential part of treating the condition. Efficient and suitable electrolyte control can help avoid problems and enhance patient outcomes.

Important facets of rhabdomyolysis's electrolyte management comprise:

1. Monitoring Electrolyte Levels: To detect and address any imbalances, careful monitoring of electrolyte levels, such as those of potassium, phosphorus, and calcium, is necessary.

2. Correcting Hyperkalemia: Heart failure and other problems might result from hyperkalemia, a typical electrolyte anomaly in

rhabdomyolysis. Diuretics like furosemide and cation exchange resins, which can be given intravenously or through dialysis, are two possible treatments for hyperkalemia.

3. Managing Hypocalcemia: The release of negatively charged proteins and phospholipids from injured muscle cells may be linked to hypocalcemia, which can happen early in rhabdomyolysis. Calcium gluconate is one treatment option for hypocalcemia; it can be given intravenously or during dialysis.

4. Treating Hyperuricemia and Hyperphosphatemia: Common electrolyte abnormalities in rhabdomyolysis include hyperphosphatemia and hyperuricemia, which can also lead to the development of additional electrolyte imbalances. Phosphate binders, including sevelamer, can be used as treatment options to lower phosphate levels, while uricosurinol can lower uric acid levels.

5. Fluid Management: Maintaining appropriate electrolyte levels and avoiding problems

associated with fluid excess or dehydration require adequate fluid resuscitation.

To summarize, the management of electrolytes during rhabdomyolysis is a multifaceted process that necessitates vigilant observation and prompt action to avert problems and enhance patient results. To guarantee thorough management of electrolyte imbalances in rhabdomyolysis, a multidisciplinary strategy including medical professionals from different specializations is imperative.

6.3 Addressing Underlying Causes

A complicated medical disorder known as rhabdomyolysis causes skeletal muscle cells that have been harmed or wounded to dissolve quickly, releasing harmful intracellular materials into the bloodstream. Myalgia, weakness, and myoglobinuria are the three symptoms that define the illness; the most sensitive test for diagnosis is an increase in creatine kinase (CK) levels.

- Rhabdomyolysis Causes

Numerous factors can lead to rhabdomyolysis, such as:

1. Damage to muscle tissue directly
2. Toxins and drugs
3. Contaminations
4. Ischemia of the muscles
5. Metabolic and electrolyte problems
6. Genetic conditions
7. Physical strain or extended bed rest
8. States brought on by temperature, such as malignant hyperthermia and neuroleptic malignant syndrome (NMS)

- Clinical Indications

Rhabdomyolysis can cause bruising, swelling, weakening, and discomfort in the muscles. Fever, malaise, and tea-colored urine—which is typically the initial symptom—are examples of systemic symptoms. Muscle soreness and other symptoms might vary greatly in intensity.

- Problems with Rhabdomyolysis

The following are the primary rhabdomyolysis complications:

1. Acute renal failure: Associated with high morbidity and mortality, this potentially fatal consequence affects up to 15% of patients. It is brought on by ischemia, renal vasoconstriction, and myoglobin's direct toxicity to the proximal convoluted tubule epithelial cells.

2. Disorders related to electrolytes: these are hypomagnesemia, hyperphosphatemia, hyperkalemia, and early hypocalcemia.

3. Coagulation disorders: A late consequence of rhabdomyolysis may be diffuse intravascular coagulation.

4. Acute respiratory distress syndrome (ARDS): Patients with underlying lung disorders or those exposed to irritants are more susceptible to this consequence, which is linked to rhabdomyolysis.

5. Multiple organ failure: Damage to the kidneys, heart, and liver, among other organs, can result from severe rhabdomyolysis.

- Identification and Management

Timely identification and management of rhabdomyolysis are essential to avert serious consequences. Laboratory testing demonstrating increased CK levels confirms the diagnosis, which is based on the patient's medical history, clinical signs, and symptoms. Correcting fluid and electrolyte imbalances and treating the underlying cause of the disease are the main goals of treatment. Patients with metabolic acidosis and potentially fatal hyperkalemia may occasionally require dialysis.

To sum up, in order to avoid complications and enhance patient outcomes, treating the underlying causes of rhabdomyolysis is essential. Health care providers can identify and treat rhabdomyolysis more accurately if they have a good awareness of the clinical signs and complications of the disorder.

Chapter Seven

Prognosis and Long-Term Effects

The rhabdomyolysis prognosis is largely influenced by the underlying etiology and related comorbidities. Rhabdomyolysis has a great prognosis when treated promptly and early, according to case reports and limited retrospective studies, despite the absence of well-organized prospective studies in this area. Additionally, there is a very good chance that the entire renal function will recover.

On the other hand, the prognosis varies greatly and is dependent upon the underlying causes and complications. Rhabdomyolysis patients have an overall mortality rate of about 5%; however, each patient's risk of death varies according to the underlying etiology and any coexisting comorbidities. The present treatment techniques' implementation has decreased morbidity and mortality. Merely 13 out of 191 (6%) patients in a 10-year retrospective pediatric evaluation passed away.

Recurrent episodes of rhabdomyolysis, particularly in youngsters, can be a long-term consequence of rhabdomyolysis and may be a sign of underlying problems in muscle structure or metabolism. It was discovered that 15% of patients had chronic renal disease (CKD) before discharge and 10% had CKD after a year in a multicenter retrospective analysis of 387 patients conducted in France. Additionally, the study discovered a correlation between admission serum myoglobin levels and long-term renal decline.

In conclusion, the underlying etiology and related comorbidities have a significant impact on the prognosis of rhabdomyolysis. Rhabdomyolysis has a great prognosis when treated aggressively and early, and full renal function can be fully recovered. The prognosis, however, varies greatly and is dependent upon the underlying causes and consequences. Recurrent episodes of rhabdomyolysis and chronic renal disease are two possible long-term complications of rhabdomyolysis.

7.1 Recovery Timeline

The degree of the illness, the underlying cause, and the course of treatment all affect how long it takes to recover from rhabdomyolysis. Recovery can be broken down into multiple stages:

1. Initial recovery: Following rhabdomyolysis therapy, a large number of patients recover, although the majority continue to have muscle weakness for a few weeks following the injury.

2. Acute kidney injury: Acute kidney injury occurs in up to 50% of cases with rhabdomyolysis. If kidney function is impaired, patients may need long-term dialysis.

3. Rehabilitation: In order to restore strength and movement, patients may need physical therapy and rehabilitation following the initial phase of recovery. Depending on how severe the muscular injury is, this procedure may take weeks to months.

4. Long-term recovery: Some patients, particularly youngsters, may have recurring

bouts of rhabdomyolysis, which may point to underlying problems with muscle structure or metabolism. 10% of patients with rhabdomyolysis after a year had chronic kidney disease (CKD), compared to 15% at the time of discharge.

In conclusion, the length of time it takes to recover from rhabdomyolysis varies greatly and is influenced by the severity of the illness, its underlying cause, and the type of treatment that is given. Although a large number of individuals make a full recovery, some may develop persistent problems and recurring bouts of rhabdomyolysis.

7.2 Potential Renal Implications

One medical disorder called rhabdomyolysis can cause acute kidney damage (AKI), among its many consequences. An increase in free ionized calcium in the cytoplasm, which impairs normal skeletal muscle action, is the pathophysiology of rhabdomyolysis. The mechanical blockage of tubules by myoglobin precipitation, the direct toxic action of free chelatable iron on tubules, and hypovolemia are the most frequent causes of AKI in rhabdomyolysis. 15% to 50% of rhabdomyolysis complications have been documented to have AKI, and this number is larger in patients who also have sepsis, dehydration, and creatine kinase levels above 15,000 IU/L (250 mckay/L).

The degree of AKI in cases of rhabdomyolysis varies greatly and is contingent upon the underlying cause and degree of muscle injury. 15% of patients with chronic kidney disease (CKD) at discharge and 10% with CKD at one year were included in a multicenter retrospective study of 387 patients conducted in France. Additionally, the study discovered a correlation between admission serum myoglobin levels and long-term renal decline.

Because severe disease can result in an accumulation of nitrogenous products in the blood (azotemia), with or without a loss in renal function and electrolyte abnormalities, prompt detection and treatment of rhabdomyolysis are essential. Resolving fluid and electrolyte imbalances and treating the underlying cause of the disorder are the mainstays of rhabdomyolysis treatment. Patients with metabolic acidosis and potentially fatal hyperkalemia may occasionally require dialysis.

To sum up, rhabdomyolysis can result in a number of issues, including AKI. The degree of muscle injury and the underlying etiology determine how severe AKI is in cases of rhabdomyolysis. Timely identification and management of rhabdomyolysis are essential to avert serious consequences. Restoring electrolyte and fluid balances and treating the underlying cause of the ailment are the mainstays of rhabdomyolysis treatment.

Chapter Eight

Prevention Strategies

The main goal of rhabdomyolysis prevention measures is to find and treat the underlying causes in order to reduce the likelihood of muscle damage and the problems that come with it. Among the most important preventative actions are:

1. Hydration: Keeping up a sufficient fluid intake can help prevent dehydration and lower the risk of muscular injury, particularly during intense physical activity.

2. Gradual activity: You can help prevent muscle overexertion and eventual damage by gradually increasing the intensity of your activity and allowing for enough rest periods.

3. Medication Monitoring: Medical professionals should closely monitor the usage of pharmaceuticals that are known to have the potential to cause rhabdomyolysis, such as

statins and some antipsychotics, and, if necessary, look into alternative treatments.

4. Awareness and Education: Early identification and intervention can be aided by educating people, especially athletes and military personnel, about the symptoms and signs of rhabdomyolysis and the significance of getting medical assistance if they feel muscle pain, weakness, or black urine.

To sum up, the prevention of rhabdomyolysis involves taking steps like drinking enough water, gradually increasing physical activity, keeping an eye on medication intake, and educating people about the need to identify and treat underlying causes in order to lower the chance of muscle damage and the consequences that come with it.

8.1 Identifying High-Risk Situations

Recognizing high-risk circumstances in rhabdomyolysis is essential to halting the progression of the illness and any consequences that may arise. Among the high-risk circumstances are:

1. "Extreme physical exertion": Excessive physical activity can cause muscular injury and rhabdomyolysis, particularly in persons who are not trained.

2. Heatstroke: Extended exposure to high temperatures can result in rhabdomyolysis and muscular damage.

3. Abuse of drugs and alcohol: Abuse of alcohol and several medications, including statins and some antipsychotics, can raise the risk of rhabdomyolysis.

4. Trauma: Rhabdomyolysis and muscle injury can result from trauma, such as crush injuries.

5. illnesses: Rhabdomyolysis and muscle injury can result from some illnesses, including influenza and viral myositis.

6. Genetic problems: Rhabdomyolysis can be more likely in people with specific genetic illnesses, including McArdle disease and myoadenylate deaminase deficiency.

7. Electrolyte imbalances: Rhabdomyolysis risk might be elevated by electrolyte imbalances, such as hypophosphatemia and hypokalemia.

In conclusion, recognizing high-risk circumstances in rhabdomyolysis is essential to halting the illness's progression and any consequences that may arise. Extreme physical exertion, heatstroke, drug and alcohol addiction, trauma, infections, genetic abnormalities, and electrolyte imbalances are examples of high-risk scenarios. Healthcare professionals who treat high-risk patients should be aware of these risk factors and take the necessary precautions to prevent rhabdomyolysis.

8.2 Exercise-Induced Rhabdomyolysis Prevention

Acute renal failure and other problems can arise from exercise-induced rhabdomyolysis (exRML), a pathophysiological disease characterized by skeletal muscle cell damage. The actions listed below can be taken to stop exRML:

1. Introduction to the Gradual Exercise: As you ease into the new exercise routine, start out slowly and steadily to give your muscles time to adjust. When your don't have enough time to recover from an intense workout, starting an exercise regimen too quickly can result in rhabdomyolysis.

2. Resist excessive activity: Excessive or severe exercise that surpasses one's physical or personal limitations may result in exRML. It's crucial to pay attention to your body's signals and cease exercising if you start to feel weak, swollen, or experience muscle pain.

3. Appropriate hydration: Make sure you consume enough fluids prior to, during, and

following exercise to avoid dehydration, which can exacerbate exRML and cause muscular damage.

4. Recovery and rest: Especially if you're new to exercising or starting a new exercise regimen, give your muscles enough time to relax and heal in between workouts.

5. Observe your symptoms: Keep an eye out for any indications of exRML, such as muscle soreness, weakness, edema, or dark urine. See a doctor right away if you experience any of these symptoms.

6. Consult a healthcare professional: Before beginning a new fitness program, make sure you are well enough to engage in the activities and talk about any possible dangers or concerns with a healthcare professional.

To summarize, the management of exercise-induced rhabdomyolysis includes introducing exercise gradually, avoiding overexertion, maintaining adequate hydration, rest, and recuperation, keeping an eye on symptoms, and seeking medical advice prior to beginning a new exercise regimen.

Chapter Nine

Case Studies and Clinical Examples

Rhabdomyolysis Case Studies and Clinical Examples

- First Case Study

After playing a high-intensity sports activity, a 28-year-old male patient arrives at the emergency room with acute muscle pain, weakness, and dark urine. His increased creatine kinase levels and the presence of myoglobin in his urine led to the diagnosis of rhabdomyolysis. After receiving intravenous fluids and electrolyte replacement, he felt better in a few days. This case emphasizes how crucial it is to be properly hydrated and introduce exercise gradually in order to prevent rhabdomyolysis, particularly in young, healthy people.

A 55-year-old woman is brought to the hospital with signs of renal failure, seizures, and disorientation. It was discovered that she has hyperkalemia and that her kidneys are not operating correctly. She gradually gets better after starting dialysis and receiving treatment for her underlying illnesses, but she continues to have recurrent episodes of rhabdomyolysis, which may indicate an underlying muscular disorder. This instance highlights the possibility of underlying muscular disorders being linked to rhabdomyolysis and highlights the significance of taking hereditary and other predisposing factors into account while managing the condition.

A 70-year-old man is taken to the hospital, exhibiting signs of exhaustion, weakness, and dyspnea. He's had diabetes, hypertension, and chronic kidney disease in the past. As his kidney function declines, rhabdomyolysis-related acute renal damage is identified as the cause of his injury. Dialysis and other supportive therapies are used to treat him, but his condition does not get better, necessitating long-term dialysis. This example emphasizes the significance of closely monitoring and managing underlying diseases as well as the potential repercussions of rhabdomyolysis in individuals with pre-existing kidney illness.

- Fourth Case Study

After engaging in an extended workout, a 19-year-old male patient arrives at the emergency room experiencing excruciating pain and cramping in his muscles. His increased creatine kinase levels and the presence of myoglobin in his urine led to the diagnosis of rhabdomyolysis. After receiving intravenous fluids and electrolyte replacement, he felt better in a few days. This case highlights how crucial it is to stay properly hydrated and get enough sleep to avoid rhabdomyolysis, particularly for people who exercise for extended periods of time.

Finally, these case reports highlight the significance of appropriate care and preventative techniques, as well as the range of clinical symptoms and problems associated with rhabdomyolysis. Aside from staying hydrated, identifying high-risk circumstances and treating underlying diseases can help avoid rhabdomyolysis and its sequelae.

9.1 Real-life scenarios illustrating clinical manifestations and complications.

Healthcare practitioners can gain a better understanding of rhabdomyolysis and its management by referring to real-life events that illustrate the condition's clinical signs and implications. Here are a few instances:

Case 1: Following his participation in a marathon, a 25-year-old male patient arrives at the emergency room with acute muscle pain, weakness, and dark urine. His increased creatine kinase levels and the presence of myoglobin in his urine led to the diagnosis of rhabdomyolysis. After receiving intravenous fluids and electrolyte replacement, he feels better in a few days. This instance emphasizes how crucial it is to be properly hydrated and introduce exercise gradually in order to prevent rhabdomyolysis, particularly in people who are engaging in continuous physical activity.

2. Case 2: Confusion, seizures, and renal failure symptoms are brought to the emergency room by a 45-year-old female patient. It was discovered that she has hyperkalemia and that her kidneys are not operating correctly. She gradually gets better after starting dialysis and receiving treatment for her underlying illnesses, but she continues to have recurrent episodes of rhabdomyolysis, which may indicate an underlying muscular disorder. This instance highlights the possibility of underlying muscular disorders being linked to rhabdomyolysis and highlights the significance of taking hereditary and other predisposing factors into account while managing the condition.

3. Case 3: Following a high-intensity workout, a 60-year-old man complains of excruciating muscle cramps and agony in the emergency room. His increased creatine kinase levels and the presence of myoglobin in his urine led to the diagnosis of rhabdomyolysis. Intravenous fluids and electrolyte replacement are used to treat him, but as his health worsens, severe renal damage occurs. His kidney function does not improve, and he needs long-term dialysis in addition to other supportive measures. The possible consequences of rhabdomyolysis are brought to light by this instance, particularly for individuals who already have kidney disease.

Case 4: Following a high-intensity workout, a 30-year-old male patient arrives at the emergency room with acute muscle soreness and weakness. His increased creatine kinase levels and the presence of myoglobin in his urine led to the diagnosis of rhabdomyolysis. After receiving intravenous fluids and electrolyte replacement, he feels better in a few days. He does, however, frequently develop rhabdomyolysis, which may indicate an underlying muscular disorder. This instance highlights how crucial it is to locate and treat underlying causes in order to stop rhabdomyolysis episodes from happening again.

In conclusion, real-world examples of rhabdomyolysis's clinical signs and consequences can aid medical practitioners in their understanding of the illness and how to treat it. Aside from staying hydrated, identifying high-risk circumstances and treating underlying diseases can help avoid rhabdomyolysis and its sequelae.

Chapter Ten

Research and Emerging Trends

The goal of rhabdomyolysis research and new trends is to comprehend the etiology, diagnosis, and treatment of the disorder. Among the principal areas of interest are:

1. Etiological classification: Direct injury to muscle tissue, medications and toxins, infections, muscle ischemia, electrolyte and metabolic disorders, genetic disorders, strenuous activity or extended bed rest, and temperature-induced conditions like neuroleptic malignant syndrome (NMS) and malignant hyperthermia are some of the factors that can lead to rhabdomyolysis.

2. Risk factors and population subgroups: Studies have been done to find population subgroups and risk factors that are more prone to rhabdomyolysis, with an emphasis on hereditary enzyme deficits and trauma.

3. Diagnosis: Because there are several possible etiologies and non-specific symptoms, diagnosing rhabdomyolysis can be difficult. On the other hand, current studies have looked into the application of imaging methods and biomarkers to increase diagnostic precision.

4. Treatment: Treating the underlying cause of rhabdomyolysis along with addressing fluid and electrolyte imbalances are the mainstays of managing the condition. Studies have been carried out to assess the efficacy of diverse therapeutic approaches and to pinpoint possible enhancements in patient results.

5. Complications: Acute kidney damage (AKI), hypoalbuminemia, hyperuricemia, compartment syndrome, and electrolyte abnormalities are among the complications of rhabdomyolysis. Studies have been carried out to gain a deeper comprehension of these issues and to create plans for managing and preventing them.

6. Prognosis: The underlying etiology and related comorbidities have a significant impact on the prognosis of rhabdomyolysis. To support clinical decision-making, research has been done to determine prognostic indicators and create risk-stratification instruments.

To sum up, studies and new developments in rhabdomyolysis are concentrated on comprehending the pathophysiology, diagnosis, and treatment of the illness, encompassing etiological categorization, risk factors, diagnostics, therapy, complications, and prognosis. The diagnosis, treatment, and prognosis of rhabdomyolysis patients can all be enhanced by these new discoveries.

10.1 Current studies and ongoing research related to rhabdomyolysis

The mechanism, diagnosis, treatment, and epidemiology of rhabdomyolysis are the main areas of interest for both recent and continuing research. The following are some current study trends and findings:

1. Pathophysiology and Diagnosis: Studies have been done to enhance the diagnosis of rhabdomyolysis and to gain a deeper understanding of its pathophysiology. This includes figuring out possible sources of muscle injury and creating more precise diagnostic techniques to find rhabdomyolysis early on.

2. Therapeutics and Management: Research has concentrated on addressing the underlying cause of rhabdomyolysis as well as assessing the efficacy of various therapeutic techniques, including fluid and electrolyte replacement. The creation of fresh management techniques to enhance patient outcomes has also been studied.

3. Epidemiology and Risk Factors: Current studies have attempted to determine which demographic subgroups are more prone to rhabdomyolysis, in addition to figuring out the main causes and risk factors of the illness. This entails looking at the prevalence of rhabdomyolysis in various patient groups as well as figuring out possible triggers and risk factors.

4. Complications and Prognosis: Research has been done to learn more about the long-term prognosis and complications of rhabdomyolysis, especially in individuals who have comorbidities. This entails assessing how rhabdomyolysis affects kidney function, the onset of chronic kidney disease, and any additional systemic side effects connected to the illness.

In summary, the goals of current research on rhabdomyolysis are to better understand the pathophysiology of the disorder, enhance diagnostic techniques, assess treatment options, pinpoint risk factors, and comprehend long-term consequences and prognoses. The goal of these research projects is to enhance rhabdomyolysis patients' diagnosis, treatment, and prognosis.

Conclusion

Recap of Key Points

The following are the salient features of rhabdomyolysis, including its clinical symptoms and complications:

1. Clinical Manifestations: Localized symptoms including bruising, swelling, weakness, and discomfort in the muscles are common in cases of rhabdomyolysis. Fever, malaise, and black urine are examples of systemic symptoms. Acute kidney damage, altered electrolyte levels, and disseminated intravascular coagulation are among the conditions' early and late complications.

2. Complications: Acute kidney injury (AKI), hypoalbuminemia, hyperuricemia, compartment syndrome, and electrolyte abnormalities are among the consequences of rhabdomyolysis. Patients with rhabdomyolysis have an overall mortality rate of about 5%, and their chance of dying depends on their underlying cause of illness as well as any coexisting conditions.

3. Diagnosis and Management: Clinical and laboratory results are used to diagnose rhabdomyolysis. The main focus of management is addressing abnormalities related to fluids and electrolytes. Particularly in children, recurrent bouts of rhabdomyolysis may be a sign of underlying problems with muscle structure or metabolism.

4. Prevention and Treatment: Strategies for preventing rhabdomyolysis include introducing exercise gradually, avoiding excessive exercise, staying properly hydrated, taking time off, recuperating from injuries, keeping an eye on symptoms, and speaking with a healthcare provider before beginning a new exercise regimen. In order to treat the condition, the underlying cause must be addressed, and any fluid and electrolyte imbalances must be corrected.

To sum up, rhabdomyolysis is a dangerous illness that can cause both local and systemic symptoms. It can also lead to potentially fatal side effects, including acute renal injury and abnormal electrolyte levels. Improving patient outcomes and lowering the risk of recurrence requires early detection, appropriate care, and preventive actions.

Importance of Timely Diagnosis and Intervention

Because of the potentially fatal consequences of rhabdomyolysis, prompt identification and treatment are essential. Early detection and treatment of rhabdomyolysis is essential since it is frequently underdiagnosed and can result in acute kidney damage, electrolyte imbalances, and systemic complications.

It is important to have a high index of suspicion and seek rapid diagnostic examination because the condition's non-specific symptoms, various etiologies, and systemic consequences make identification difficult. With 26,000 instances reported annually in the US, rhabdomyolysis is a prevalent ailment in adult populations. Therefore, prompt identification is crucial to avoiding the associated morbidity and mortality.

The American Association for the Surgery of Trauma's clinical consensus document highlights the importance of current rhabdomyolysis diagnosis, treatment, and prognosis. It also emphasizes the need for useful answers to frequently asked clinical questions that are based on expert consensus and a literature review.

One of the most crucial treatment objectives when rhabdomyolysis is suspected is to prevent acute kidney damage, highlighting the need for prompt diagnosis and intervention to avert serious consequences.

In summary, life-threatening consequences, including acute renal injury and electrolyte imbalances, can be avoided by promptly diagnosing and treating rhabdomyolysis. Healthcare practitioners should maintain a high index of suspicion and swiftly commence diagnostic and therapeutic steps when rhabdomyolysis is suspected, given the condition's underdiagnosis and severe systemic consequences.

Reference

Bosch, X., Poch, E., & Grau, J. M. (2015). Rhabdomyolysis and acute kidney injury. The New England Journal of Medicine, 372(18), 1750-1750. https://doi.org/10.1056/NEJMc1500961

Burgess, S. (2022). Rhabdomyolysis: An evidence-based approach. Sage Journals. https://doi.org/10.1177/17511437211050782

Huerta-Alardín, A. L., Varon, J., & Marik, P. E. (2014). Bench-to-bedside review: Rhabdomyolysis – an overview for clinicians. Critical Care, 18(3), 1-10. https://doi.org/10.1186/cc13862

Singh, U., Scheld, W. M., & Kumar, A. (2015). Rhabdomyolysis: Pathogenesis, diagnosis, and treatment. Clinical Infectious Diseases, 62(1), 146-153. https://doi.org/10.1093/cid/civ773

UpToDate. (2022). Rhabdomyolysis: Clinical manifestations and diagnosis. https://www.uptodate.com/contents/rhabdomyolysis-clinical-manifestations-and-diagnosis

About the Author

Dr. Robert Neil is a distinguished author and veteran researcher in the field of rhabdomyolysis. His extensive contributions have significantly advanced the understanding of the clinical manifestations, complications, diagnosis, and management of this complex medical condition. Dr. Neil's research has been instrumental in shedding light on the etiology and frequency of rhabdomyolysis, as well as providing an evidence-based approach to the diagnosis and management of this underdiagnosed and life-threatening complication. His work has been published in reputable journals and has been widely recognized for its impact on clinical practice and patient care.

Dr. Neil's publication, "Rhabdomyolysis: An evidence-based approach," provides a comprehensive overview of the condition, emphasizing the importance of timely diagnosis and intervention. His research has also been instrumental in developing clinical consensus documents that review the present-day diagnosis, management, and prognosis of rhabdomyolysis, providing practical answers to common clinical questions based on expert consensus and literature review. Dr. Neil's dedication to addressing the pathogenesis, diagnosis, and treatment of rhabdomyolysis has significantly contributed to the advancement of medical knowledge in this field.

Overall, Dr. Robert Neil's work has made a significant impact on the field of rhabdomyolysis, and his contributions continue to be invaluable for healthcare professionals, researchers, and patients alike.